MOMENTS OF VICTORY, MOMENTS OF CHANGE:
Stories of Perseverance and Quiet Courage

Dorothy Hill Baroch, M.A.

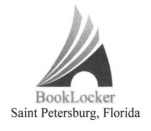

BookLocker
Saint Petersburg, Florida

ISBN: 978-1-64718-819-1

Published by BookLocker.com, Inc., St. Petersburg, Florida.

Printed on acid-free paper.

BookLocker.com, Inc.
2020

First Edition

Library of Congress Cataloging in Publication Data
Baroch, M.A., Dorothy Hill
MOMENTS OF VICTORY, MOMENTS OF CHANGE: Stories of Perseverance and Quiet Courage by Dorothy Hill Baroch, M.A.
Library of Congress Control Number: 2020917154

To Tom Baroch

I dedicate this book to our son, Tom,
an advocate for those fighting battles
against life–threatening ailments.
His strength and courage bring hope
to people around the world.

The life stories presented in the book
tell the tales of his actions
and those of other heroes
who have fought and conquered
unbelievable challenges.

May their hard work inspire others
to do the same.

ACKNOWLEDGEMENTS

Countless emails flew across cyberspace over the years as I pursued a dream, a dream of recognizing and acknowledging fascinating individuals–some I had met face to face, others through the world of technology, others through the recollections of family members. As their stories unfolded, my vision grew, and what was once only the nugget of an idea eventually became a reality. Concepts came and went, like the shifting sand, until a solid plan began to form and the initial outline for *Moments of Victory, Moments of Change* was put on paper.

As I learned of the courage and persistence of other people, new names were added to my list: those sometimes forgotten or overlooked individuals who haven't met society's standards for success. Yet success is what every one of the people in the book has accomplished. They are victorious and triumphant, humble and courageous–people I have come to know, to love, and to have a great desire to emulate.

You will meet many of my heroes and heroines as you turn the pages–people who have displayed endless courage and persistence during the uphill battle of life. Obstacles blocked their paths–sometimes for a few days, sometimes for months, sometimes for years–but inevitably their tenacity won out. To each individual and family in this book, I offer my deepest gratitude.

Some of my heroes and heroines you *will not* meet in the pages of *Moments of Victory, Moments of Change*. They are the people whose dedication to words and story line, grammar and punctuation, publication guidelines and details helped me accomplish my goal of writing a book about hope.

I offer a huge thank you and my deepest appreciation to:

My dear husband, Ed, and my children, Steve, Vickie and Mary, who lived *Tom's Story* with me, and who continually encouraged me as I walked the writing journey that I hope will bring enlightenment to my readers;

Dr. James R. (Jim) Welsh, former neighbor, friend, and computer guru who had the patience and dedication to change margins and adjust fonts endlessly, and to organize the book into a system acceptable to the publisher;

Deanna Campbell, miracle worker par excellence, whose insight and skill with the "red pen" brought polish to the manuscript;

Kathy Price–Toby, who lovingly volunteered her talent as a copy editor to this project;

The staff and members of the Spina Bifida Association, for their tireless efforts to build a better and brighter future for all those impacted by this permanently disabling birth defect;

Finally, to members of the Wenatchee Valley Writers Group in Washington state and the Sun City Writers Group in Las Vegas, Nevada–a collection of dedicated writers who supported me, guided me and often corrected me–always with the intent of helping me to create a product of value. Though more than one thousand miles apart, geographically, they are of the same heart and mind.

ABOUT THE AUTHOR

Dorothy Hill Baroch, wife, mother of four, and author, entered the disability world in 1959, when her son, Tom, was born with Spina Bifida and hydrocephalus. The family's journey brought them into contact with other people who also encountered incredible medical and psychological challenges–people who sought the best possible solutions in a world that often was ignorant of their needs. Baroch watched as accessibility awareness grew, medical progress was made, and people with Spina Bifida began to live beyond the normal early childhood death. The life stories of some of those affected by Spina Bifida are presented in Part I of *Moments of Victory*. Part II presents stories of people who have found the courage to face and conquer other types of disabilities.

Baroch lives with her husband, Ed, in Summerlin, a suburb of Las Vegas, Nevada. She has traveled extensively, and besides her writing efforts, enjoys reading, embroidering, and visiting with family members. In addition to *Moments of Victory, Moments of Change*, Baroch wrote and published *Listen to the Heartbeat of the Church* and authored numerous magazine articles.

Sara Struwe, MPA

President and Chief Executive Officer
Spina Bifida Association

Spina Bifida, which literally means split spine, is a complex birth defect that occurs in the first four weeks of pregnancy. When the spine is forming, the spine does not "zip up" correctly, and there is a gap left that exposes the spinal cord throughout a pregnancy.

What happens next depends on so many things–where the lesion on the spine occurs, the care the person receives, the family he or she is born into, and others. Some people walk with minimal noticeable issues, others depend on a wheelchair, some may use crutches, and some will use a variety of these methods to get from one place to another in their lives. Most will have trouble using the bathroom on their own and will depend on bowel management programs and clean intermittent catheterization. Some will have hydrocephalus and will require a shunt in their brains to drain excess fluid, and they will face many brain surgeries in their lives.

Others may face social isolation that comes with a condition like Spina Bifida. In general, the world doesn't understand that being different is okay, and they look at people as broken who walk differently or use a wheelchair to get around. This often leaves people feeling lonely and sometimes in despair.

But despite all of this, people with Spina Bifida bring a light to this world. Their stories are complex, funny, moving, and sometimes, dare I say, inspiring–not because they do normal things that everyone does, but because they move mountains.

While Spina Bifida used to be considered a childhood disease, people now live well into old age. It is estimated that more than 65% of the people living with Spina Bifida are adults. They are doctors, attorneys, teachers, nurses, social workers, and advocates, among other work. They get married and have children, and grandchildren, thanks to the fact that their childhood care has improved so much.

Spina Bifida is often referred to as a snowflake condition because no two cases of Spina Bifida are the same. But the truth is that the people are the real snowflakes, in the best positive way. They indeed are unique individuals who give so much to those who take the time to get to know them.

This book tells the stories of a few individuals in the Spina Bifida community as well as people dealing with addiction and Alzheimer's. It shines a light on their truth, their light, and what they bring to this world. I hope that you will enjoy their stories and get to know some of my dear friends.

Table of Contents

MOMENTS OF VICTORY, MOMENTS OF CHANGE:
Stories of Perseverance and Quiet Courage

INTRODUCTION

Moments of Victory, Moments of Change is a collection of life stories, a glimpse into the minds and hearts of individuals and families who faced, and in some cases continue to face, adversity with faith and determination. While the stories are different, threads of hope and courage are woven throughout, connecting them, and forming a common bond. Each chapter contains the story of an individual or family and their accomplishments in the face of difficult conditions, medical or emotional issues, or other hardships.

The intent is to honor the tenacity of the people and their families who have willingly shared their stories and to express appreciation for the communities of love and support that surround them.

Napoleon Hill, an American self–help author, once said, "Strength and growth come only through continuous effort and struggle."

The life stories in *Moments of Victory, Moments of Change* are about individuals who face, struggle with, and move beyond major challenges. It is a book about hope and determination.

PART ONE
The World of Spina Bifida

A Tribute to Tom Baroch
By Jesus Arroyo

"There are people that fight for a day, and they are good...
"There are people that fight for a few years, and they are better...
"There are people that fight their entire lives, those people are vital."

I saw these words on the wall of a building in Guatemala my first time there. And they remind me of my friend. He fought his entire life, for his own survival, and for the survival of others with Spina Bifida...for their quality of life, for health care, and so they wouldn't be forgotten.

I will miss you my friend.

Thomas Edmund Baroch
December 13, 1959–November 4, 2018

CHAPTER ONE

Tom's Story:
A Passionate Disability Advocate
Dorothy Hill Baroch

I first met Thomas (Tom) Baroch in the summer of 1959, when I was a few months pregnant with him. My husband, Ed, and I were asleep in our camp tent, nestled among the trees of an orchard in Central Oregon, when I felt–for the first time–movement in my womb. I woke Ed and told him the motion felt like the wings of a butterfly–gently letting me know our first child was growing and ready to be noticed.

On December 14 of that same year, less than twenty–four hours after Tom's birth, he slept peacefully in the nursery of Albany, Oregon's General Hospital, unaware of the future chaos and challenges he, and our family, would face. Down the hall, in the maternity ward, I was in tears. The doctor had given orders that I could not hold my son, the nurse said, "because he has some problems that Dr. O'Neill will discuss with you." Thoughts, queries and worries roiled through my brain. *What could be wrong?*

Exhausted from a long labor and difficult delivery, I eventually fell asleep. When I awakened, the nurse told me Dr. O'Neill would like to talk with me. I watched him saunter down the hall, stop at my doorway, and knock. He leaned against the door frame, seemingly unable to step across the threshold. "Dorothy," he said, "your baby has a major birth defect, and probably will not live. If he does, more than likely he will become a vegetable. I recommend that you and Ed put him in an institution and go about raising the rest of your family."

After some questions on my part, the doctor explained that Tom was born with Spina Bifida (myelomeningocele) and probably hydrocephalus. His spine had not closed properly and there was a sac with nerve endings protruding through the opening of the spinal column. He said that this situation would undoubtedly create multiple problems throughout his life, if he lived at all. I listened attentively, trying to absorb words and concepts that were completely unfamiliar to me. With tears streaming down my cheeks, I looked at the doctor and said, "Thank you for the advice, Dr. O'Neill, but Tom is a gift from God and belongs with us. We're taking him home. Will you help us?"

That began the first thread of advocacy, a thread which would be woven into a tapestry of love, support, and service within and beyond our family, a tapestry that would spread across four continents.

How did we, parents in our early twenties, cope with raising a child who required major surgeries, repeated doctors' visits, and a constant, watchful eye? Ed was a young father and husband, beginning his career as a metallurgical engineer. I was a twenty–two–year–old mother, living 3,000 miles from her parents and sister. Out of necessity, we learned to seek and ask for the support our new, young family needed. Friends from our church became like family. Workmates of Ed were helpful and caring.

We were determined to seek the best medical advice and guidance we could. Phone calls to doctors and medical facilities, and questions addressed to friends and sometimes strangers, opened one door after another, as we began what seemed at times, to be a career in advocacy. Eventually, we built a medical team that saw us through surgeries, frustrations, and the challenges which come to a family that deals with physical disabilities.

Ed and I had two more children, Steve and Vickie, who were healthy. We eventually adopted a third, Mary Frances, from Korea. After Tom's birth, we had decided to make our family life as normal as possible. We did not coddle Tom; we accommodated his problems but didn't allow them to overshadow his talents and abilities. We traveled, went on family camping trips, taught him to ride a bike, and allowed him to play any of the games he felt he could play. Ed even bought him a Pogo stick. While that may have been a mistake, since Tom's balance was not good, it was another normalizing act–a statement that he was "just a kid."

Eventually, we involved Tom in making decisions about his health care and taught him to advocate for himself. We encouraged him to seek advice from competent people, primarily his physicians, and to work with us in making important decisions about his health and day–to–day activities. At age ten, and after discussion with his orthopedic doctor, Tom was emphatic about his desire not to wear the leg braces he had on for seven years. The leg braces of today are made of light metal and plastic, with lightweight rivets and screws. Tom's braces were made of a heavier steel or brass, foam, and heavyweight leather to cover the foam. They were cumbersome and stiff, limiting movement, which is what they were supposed to do. Tom complained about the braces because he *knew* he was capable of more leg movement without them. One day he confided, "I quietly tested this at night after I had taken them off for the day and no one was watching. Looking back, I think that was pretty sneaky and smart for a 10–year–old!" The braces were discarded!

During junior high and high school, which were relatively normal, he came to grips with what his disability really was and how to deal with it, both physically and socially. He delivered newspapers for the Albany Democrat–Herald and worked as a line cook for the local A&W restaurant. From sixth grade through high school, yearly, all–day trips to visit a Spina Bifida clinic in Portland, Oregon were informative but demanding. He was active in the Albany, Oregon Columbian Squires (Junior Knights of Columbus) and served a term as president. Tom enjoyed the outdoors and participated in a Junior Search and Rescue program through the Linn County Sheriff's office in Oregon.

Self–advocacy became part of his life. His sojourn at a prep school, located fifty miles from our home, provided opportunities for maturing. Like his young mother years ago, he didn't have immediate family at his beck and call. After some trial and error, however, Tom learned to ask for help, to make his own decisions, and to carve his own path. That path led to self–determination, which Pacer's National Parent Center on Transition and Employment describes as "…a combination of attitudes and abilities that lead people to set goals for themselves, and to take the initiative to reach these goals. It is about being in charge but is not necessarily the same thing as self–sufficiency or independence. It means making your own choices, learning to effectively solve problems, and taking control and responsibility for one's life. Practicing self–determination also means one experiences the consequences of making choices."[1]

Tom took a year between high school and college to work and travel. He applied to, and was accepted by, the University of Nevada Reno and Arizona State University with a goal of being a Physical Therapist. For a number of reasons, he chose Reno, most importantly, because it was his father's alma mater and it was closer to home. He lived in Lincoln Hall, the same residence hall in which his father had lived and was Dorm President–receiving an award as an Outstanding Residence Hall Student. After his first semester, he found that he was geared more toward the humanities than math and science, and he changed his major. Once more, being away from family, living in a dorm, and making his own life–style choices offered additional options for

---

[1] http://www.pacer.org/transition/learning–center/independent–community–living/self–determination.asp.

maturity. He would say, "I was raised in Albany, Oregon; I grew up in Reno, Nevada."

After two years in Reno, he returned to the Northwest, found a job working for an accountant, saved some money, and began a two–year program at a community college in Portland, Oregon. Tom graduated with an Associate of Applied Science Degree– Sous Chef. Four years later, he attended Washington State University's School of Business, completing their Hotel and Restaurant Administration program. He received a Certificate in Conventions and Meetings Management.

Tom found his niche in the non–profit world when he attended the 1996 national Spina Bifida Conference in Phoenix, Arizona. "That was the first time as an adult that I had meaningful interaction with others directly affected by Spina Bifida. It changed my outlook as a person with a disability and motivated me to consider how I could advocate for others with disabilities." He chose to focus only on medical issues that were essential to his overall health or that made him feel physically better. "I lived life and paid as little attention to my disability as possible."

In 2000, Tom, Ed, and I attended an SBA conference in Milwaukee, Wisconsin, where we presented a session on "Living with Spina Bifida for Forty Years." In 2002 he and his father visited Guatemala, where they saw, first–hand, the disability issues in that country that stemmed from a high incidence of Spina Bifida and hydrocephalus. Tom returned a year later with grant money he had acquired through the Christopher Reeve Foundation. During his lifetime, he traveled to Guatemala more than a dozen times, providing medical equipment donations, working with Rotary Clubs, and helping to get the International Spina Bifida Conference to be held in Guatemala for the first time.

He attended every national SBA conference from 2000 through 2008. Tom expanded his advocacy efforts through his involvement in the International Federation for Spina Bifida and Hydrocephalus (IF), attending IF conferences in Poland, Norway, Finland, and Kenya.

Tom quietly touched the lives of those around him. As a little boy, he often watched from the sidelines. He once told me that he watched when others were doing things that he could not do, but only until he figured out a way to do the same thing–his way. He faced life's challenges without complaint and with fortitude. He affected people's lives worldwide, offering his skills in a variety of ways to help people with disabilities, and teaching others to help them as well. He touched my life in ways beyond measure–modeling patience, courage, and simplicity.

His professional and volunteer careers encompassed multiple aspects of the non–profit world, where his advocacy skills helped others in need. Those skills were also used to teach us, his aging parents, how to weave our way through the medical quagmire that was an integral part of his journey. Life comes full circle!

Tom died unexpectedly on November 4th, 2018 of a pulmonary embolism. He left behind a legacy of dedication and kindness, following the example of St. Teresa of Calcutta–helping the poorest of the poor, those often ignored or left by the wayside.

The image of a butterfly that I had of Tom when he was not yet born changed when he became an adult, to that of an eagle, a beautiful creature of strength and grace that he admired.

The Spina Bifida Association (SBA) established a Tom Baroch Memorial Fund page, with the following quote:

"He was a long–time advocate who worked hard to make sure that the Spina Bifida community's voices were heard both in the United States and abroad, especially in Guatemala. He served on the Spina Bifida Association's (SBA) Board of Directors from 2001 to 2004; worked intensively with the SBA of Colorado and the International Federation for Spina Bifida and Hydrocephalus; attended SBA's first annual Teal on the Hill advocacy event,

writing a reflection on his experience; and was working to help establish a Spina Bifida clinic in Las Vegas, Nevada."

A scholarship fund in Tom's name was established shortly after he died. The idea originated with the board of the SBA and their CEO, Sara Struwe. Our son, Steve, brought the idea to our family and we readily agreed that it was something Tom would have wanted. The Tom Baroch Memorial Scholarship Fund was created to allow individuals with Spina Bifida, who could not afford the cost, to attend SBA's annual advocacy event in Washington, D.C. In 2018, Tom attended the first "Teal on the Hill" (teal is the color SBA uses in their brand). In 2019, because of the generosity of family and friends, nine people ("Tom's Team" as they were named) attended because of the scholarship donations. Along with approximately 115 other people with Spina Bifida and hydrocephalus, the "Team" visited more than 75 legislators on Capitol Hill–telling their stories and asking for funding. Picture if you will, 115 people in wheelchairs and scooters, with crutches and walkers, from 27 states, navigating Capitol Hill. They requested $8 million for the National Spina Bifida Program, housed at the National Center on Birth Defects and Disabilities at the Centers for Disease Control and Prevention. As of March 2019, that request was granted by the House of Representatives Committee on Appropriations Sub–committee on Labor, Health, and Human Services in Washington, D. C. and was sent to the Senate for action.

In addition to the scholarship fund, the SBA Board created the Thomas Baroch Advocacy Award, the first one of which was given to Donna Cruz Jones, one of Tom's close friends and a friend of our family. Donna had given testimony in mid–March 2019 to the House Committee, telling of her life as an adult with Spina Bifida. She received the award at the closing dinner of the 2019 "Teal on the Hill."

Tom's physical presence is no longer with us, but his story continues, through the commitment and perseverance of his family, friends, and colleagues and through his legacy of advocacy on behalf of all those who suffer from the effects of Spina Bifida and hydrocephalus.

CHAPTER TWO

Growing Old with Spina Bifida
Donna Cruz Jones
In cooperation with Dorothy Hill Baroch

"You is smart. You is kind. You is important."

That well–known quote from the movie, *The Help*, fits Donna Cruz Jones to a "T." Donna would probably not define herself that way but, for the many friends and associates who love and respect her, it is a perfect description.

The following is an overview of Donna's life journey and includes part of her testimony to the House of Representatives Committee on Appropriations Sub–committee on Labor, Health, and Human Services in Washington, D. C. March 18, 2019.[2]

"When I was born (with Spina Bifida) on the island of Guam in 1976, the doctors told my parents, 'She will never walk, never talk, and will be a vegetable the rest of her life. You already have one healthy daughter; you should focus on her and institutionalize the other one, just walk away.'"

Thankfully, her parents ignored the doctors' advice and on April 20th, 2020, Donna celebrated her 44th birthday.

"I love birthdays because with every passing year, I defy all the negative predictions about what my life would be. I am happy to be part of the first generation of people with Spina Bifida to survive to adulthood. The biggest obstacle to surviving is that adult care doctors do not have protocols in place to treat our myriad issues. Most have never had a patient with Spina Bifida. The majority of the Spina Bifida population remains under the care of multiple pediatric specialists. These doctors are the only

---

[2] Donna's testimony has been modified from the original transcript.

ones who have treated a large number of us. I may never transition to adult care.

"Like 80% of people with myelomeningocele (the most common and most severe type of Spina Bifida), I have a pump, called a shunt, installed in my head that drains cerebral spinal fluid off my brain. My shunt is basically my second heart. I cannot live without it. Excess fluid on the brain, called hydrocephalus, is incredibly dangerous. It can lead to irreparable brain damage or death if not treated. Unfortunately, there is nothing that I can do to keep my shunt functioning. I am basically at its mercy and, if it does malfunction, I need brain surgery to have it replaced. The recovery from shunt revision is long and painful. I count myself lucky that I have only had 14 shunt revisions throughout my life. I have friends, younger than I, who have endured 50 shunt revisions. But as a result of my many shunt revisions, I have developed seizures caused by scarring on the brain. I take very powerful anti–seizure medicines to keep them under control and, I'm happy to say, this medicine is working very well.

"I don't live in fear of my Spina Bifida. The truth is, I don't sit at home bemoaning my health problems and I absolutely do not allow myself to be sorry that I have Spina Bifida. I am too busy training in Los Angeles to break the women's U. S. bench press record. The current record stands at 243 pounds; I intend to break that record with a 260–pound lift. I have a long way to go; however, I am determined to reach my goal. Finally, having used a wheelchair for more than six years, I am now taking physical therapy because I am determined to walk again.

"I don't ever want anyone to pity me. I have a wonderful life. I truly believe I am not a mistake and I was born with Spina Bifida for a reason. I'm very blessed to have had only three surgeries in the last six years. I am doing extremely well, and I love who I am as a person with a disability. I have zero regrets. That being said, I hope to see in my lifetime a cure for Spina Bifida. As much as I

love my life, I do not want another child with Spina Bifida to have 32 surgeries as I've had, or 60 surgeries like some of my friends. **No, I do not want that.**

"*My dear friend and mentor, Tom Baroch, died in November 2018 at the age of 58. I miss him more every day, but I take comfort in knowing that he didn't die of a Spina Bifida related problem. He died from a pulmonary embolism, like so many people who don't have Spina Bifida. Tom got to grow old with Spina Bifida. I know most adults don't consider 58 as old. But by Spina Bifida standards, I am old, as was Tom. My neurosurgeon jokingly tells me every time I see him, 'Now try to behave, Donna, because you're old with Spina Bifida.' He is right. I am old, but I want the opportunity to grow old enough to look in the mirror and see wrinkles on my face and more gray hairs on my head than I can count. This is a dream I never allowed myself to have until I was in my 30s.*"

During her testimony Donna clearly described the need for additional financial support, asking that the committee increase funding for the National Spina Bifida Patient Registry as well as additional funding for a hydrocephalus protocol development.

"*Under the auspices of the Centers for Disease Control and Prevention, the National Center for Birth Defects and Developmental Disabilities and the Spina Bifida Association have developed the National Spina Bifida Patient Registry. The Registry stores data on patients from twenty–four Spina Bifida clinics in the United States. Its primary purpose is to collect information on health issues patients are experiencing and the treatment they receive, which will ultimately be studied to determine the effectiveness of the treatment. My medical information is part of the Registry. My doctors at Duke University run a stellar program for treating patients with Spina Bifida. I hope my medical history will help develop sound medical treatments so people with Spina Bifida can live longer, healthier lives. Even though I live in California, I travel to the Duke University Pediatric Spina Bifida clinic to receive care. I'm lucky that I can afford this luxury."*

In her closing remarks, Donna expressed her gratitude for the opportunity to ask for additional funding and give her testimony.

"These funds will help those who come after me live healthier lives and will help us all live long enough to see wrinkles on our faces."

CHAPTER THREE

A Man of Quiet Courage:
Harold Fredrick Ridenour

Submitted by Marilyn Goodman, Marcie Goodman Stumpf, and Stacey Goodman Mihallik
Edited by Dorothy Hill Baroch

Superstars promoted in the media often overshadow the unsung heroes in our world, those individuals whose lives affect others in a subtle and understated manner. Harold Frederick Ridenour, or "Papa" as he is still referred to by his family, was one of those behind–the–scenes people. Dark–haired and of medium build, he was easy–going and handsome, according to his daughter, Marilyn. Thought to be the oldest person in the United States who lived with Spina Bifida, Harold died of natural causes on December 30, 2006, two months before his 91st birthday.

For the most part, his life was uneventful–and therein lies his story. He met the challenges of his physical disabilities as he met the challenges of his life as a farmer–with a determined attitude, a quiet demeanor, and a strong will. He lived life to the fullest, overcoming heartache and multiple disasters.

Harold was born to Marzella and Fred Ridenour on February 16, 1916, his father's birthday. The delivery took place at home, on the family farm located in southern Cedar County, Iowa, just a few miles north of West Liberty.

After the birth of their two daughters, four–year old Louise and 15–month old Lela, the Ridenours were delighted to have a son. Sadly, their joy was marred by the baby's deformity–a bag of nerves evident at the base of his spine. In that era, the condition–

myelomeningocele[3] or Spina Bifida—was a virtual death sentence. Because medical personnel had convinced them that the baby would die, the Ridenours chose not to apply for a birth certificate, something Harold didn't realize until years later when he began to travel and needed a passport.

His parents and sisters treated the tiny infant gently, knowing that if the bag of nerves ruptured, it would cause certain death. To protect him against that possibility, his mother carried him around on a pillow until, at the age of six months, he underwent surgery at the University of Iowa Hospitals and Clinics in Iowa City. The surgeons inserted the bag of nerves back into his body and closed the area successfully, a traumatic event for a child, but one that saved his life.

Harold was a healthy and happy toddler. He ran and played like any other little boy, riding his tricycle, and taking his pony, Daisy, on long jaunts.

His sister, Lela, was his main playmate during their elementary school years. She was a tomboy and the two of them played together after school, swinging on a rope in the haymow, even climbing to the top of the windmill. When Lela contracted polio at age ten, everything changed, for her and for Harold.

Although she suffered most of her life from the after–effects of that disease, Lela worked hard to surmount the difficulties caused by polio. Marzella acted as her daughter's physical therapist, making her crawl—every day—on her hands and knees

---

[3] **Myelomeningocele:** A myelomeningocele is the most serious form of spina bifida. In babies with a myelomeningocele, the bones of the spine (vertebrae) don't form properly. This lets a small sac extend through an opening in the spine. The sac is covered with a membrane. It holds cerebrospinal fluid (CSF) and tissues that protect the spinal cord (meninges). The sac may also contain portions of the spinal cord and nerves. Excerpt taken from the website of Seattle Children's Hospital: https://www.seattlechildrens.org

from the house to the barn. The child's knees were bruised and sore, but that tough love approach worked. Because of it, Lela became mobile. To her mother's credit, Lela needed only crutches, enabling her to walk rather than using a wheelchair.

When Harold started school, he discovered another disability that, in some ways, was worse than Spina Bifida. He was dyslexic[4]. "Since dyslexia was a relatively unknown condition then, my dad was considered dumb," said his daughter, Marilyn. "He had a terrible time reading and had an extremely poor sense of direction. Papa made sure there was a compass in each vehicle, so he would know where he was going.

"Aunt Lela read his lessons to him and helped him with his homework. Papa said that if it hadn't been for his sister, he wouldn't have made it through school. Both of his sisters were valedictorians of their class, so my dad must have been a disappointment to himself because he didn't achieve the same success in the classroom."

Harold regretted not being able to participate in school sports, but probably wouldn't have had the time because he had to work on the family farm. His parents did allow him to join Future Farmers of America (FFA), though. In high school, he was a charter member of the West Liberty FFA and took pride in that accomplishment, especially because the school honored him with a ceremony and a plaque later in life.

Harold's father was not very ambitious and was a tough taskmaster. Marilyn remembers that her grandfather "never cut

---

[4] **Dyslexia**: A learning disorder characterized by difficulty reading. Also called specific reading disability, dyslexia is a common learning disability in children. Dyslexia occurs in children with normal vision and intelligence. Sometimes, dyslexia goes undiagnosed for years and isn't recognized until adulthood. Excerpt taken from the Mayo Clinic website: http://www.mayoclinic.com

Dad any slack and was, at times, downright abusive in his language if his son made a mistake. Thank heavens Grandma was a real sweetheart; she tried to make amends for the things Grandpa said. I've often wondered, though, if my grandfather's actions strengthened Dad's will, which may have helped him later in life."

As a teen, Harold spent most of his time working, especially after his father retired in his 40s. "Grandpa never did a tap of work from then on," said Marilyn. "Grandma waited on him hand and foot and the rest of the family did all of the chores–shoveling snow, mowing the lawn, taking care of the animals and other farm work."

Because of the demands on his time at home, Harold's social life was limited to FFA and an occasional evening out. Marilyn remembers that he had two good high school friends and dated one girl before friends introduced him to Martha Elaine Watters, who attended high school in a neighboring town. Martha's naturally curly red hair and her bubbly personality attracted Harold, and they began dating.

After high school and one year of junior college, Martha moved to Illinois with her parents and Harold continued working on the family farm. They continued to date, beginning a long–distance courtship with Harold driving into Chicago on a regular basis. Eventually, they decided to marry and had a quiet, simple wedding on New Year's Eve 1938, at the minister's house. Their only attendants were Martha's sister, Margaret, and Harold's brother–in–law, Elmer Kline.

The young couple had no honeymoon, little money, and immediately moved to the Watters farm owned by Martha's parents. Harold's father was furious; so furious, in fact, that he wouldn't let Harold take his pony, Daisy, to the Watters acreage. Fred wanted the newlyweds to live with him and Marzella and farm the home place, allowing Fred to continue in his rather easy lifestyle.

Martha and Harold worked hard. Their life centered on family, the church, and neighborhood get–togethers. Marilyn remembers that her parents had a very strong marriage. "It was a good thing because they faced a lot of obstacles. They lost their first two children, Elaine, and David. Elaine died in the hospital when she was just two weeks old. David had a hole in his heart and lived for six weeks. They never got over the deaths, and until the day he died, Dad couldn't talk about the babies without crying." Less than a year after David's death, they adopted four–month old Ronnie and Marilyn was born three years later, in 1945.

Life on a farm meant that the children had to entertain themselves. "We had an assortment of pets," said Marilyn, "lots of cats and a little Pekinese–mix dog named Trixie. Mom raised chickens to butcher, but when they were chicks, they were fun to play with. We also had the occasional orphaned lamb that needed to be bottle–fed. We didn't learn to swim, so there were no trips to the pool in town for us."

The family wasn't close to Grandpa Fred and Grandma Marzella, so Marilyn and Ronnie didn't visit them for special play days, but "Grandma Marzella did take pity on me when Mom went to work," Marilyn recalls. "I was about junior high age, and she and Grandpa would take me shopping occasionally. But my summers were rather lonely, with Mom and Dad both working." A huge fire in the 1940s destroyed every building except the house on the Watters farm. Even though they were still renting the farm from Martha's parents, the event was traumatic. Harold helped to rebuild the structures. "That's just what tough farmers did," Marilyn said with pride.

In 1950, the couple faced yet another obstacle. Harold broke his back when a grain elevator fell on him. During the six months he was in a body cast, the family hired someone to do the farming, but that incident and his Spina Bifida surgery, resulted in constant back problems.

When Martha's parents died, the young Ridenours inherited the Watters acreage. They not only farmed that land for fifty years; they also rented another one hundred acres north of their property.

In 1956, the crops were at their peak when a huge hailstorm came through. It hit both farms, circled around, and hit them again. The crops were destroyed. To save money, Harold had not purchased hail insurance that year, and they were down to their last $200. They went to Harold's father, Fred, for help but he refused to lend them money and told them to work it out on their own. A relative of Martha's sold them corn for their livestock at a very low price, which saved the animals.

That tragedy was the beginning of Martha's working career outside of the farm and home. She found a job in Iowa City at a brush factory, now known as Oral B Products, and worked there for twenty years. Her job helped the Ridenours struggle through those tough financial times. Harold also took a job driving a grain truck to earn some extra money.

"When Mom went to work, and when Dad wasn't busy during planting and harvesting seasons, he was the housekeeper. We hated the monotonous oatmeal and Cream of Wheat breakfasts, but he insisted that we have a hearty meal in the morning," remembers Marilyn. "He packed Mom's lunch every day for twenty years, cleaned the house and even ironed, until we complained about the way he did it. That was it for the ironing."

After Martha and Harold retired in 1978, they traveled extensively, visiting Australia, New Zealand, and every state in the union except Florida. They had planned to visit Florida for a month, but Martha had her first heart attack, so they put those plans aside. They sold their house and thirty acres in 1988, keeping the rest of the farmland, and moved into West Liberty where they lived for ten years. When Martha's health began to fail, they moved to an independent living complex, their home until she died in 2001.

"Dad was lost without Mom," said Marilyn. "She had always done the bookwork, paid all the bills, and was his dearest companion for sixty–two years."

Marilyn recalls that as he aged, his leg and foot became more and more deformed, requiring him to wear a leg brace the last ten years of his life. As his health deteriorated, so did his will to live. "The last straw," said Marilyn "was not being able to drive. He was ready to die. *What was there to live for?*

"Dad was a wonderful man who didn't have an enemy in the world. At his visitation, I was told repeatedly what a good person he was–steadfast in his dedication to his family and concerned about others.

"He read everything he could about Spina Bifida, including a newspaper story about a teenager in Davenport who had the affliction. He located her phone number and called her. They talked for quite a while and Dad tried to encourage her in every way he could.

"I miss him terribly, but when I look back on his life, I realize that he was an absolute miracle."

Spina Bifida affects approximately 166,000 individuals and 3,000 pregnancies every year. People with that disability face a host of obstacles, including, but not limited to physical, developmental, educational, and vocational challenges.[5]

Harold Ridenour–not expected to live past infancy–exceeded the average life span of most people, including people without SB. He left a legacy of strength, determination, and kindness. He was a man of quiet courage.

---

[5] https://www.spinabifidaassociation.org

CHAPTER FOUR

One Tough Old Broad
Marge Hays
In cooperation with Dorothy Hill Baroch

As a septuagenarian, Marge Hays parasails, swims, boxes, snorkels, zip lines, and rides horses. That is quite an accomplishment for any able–bodied person. For a risk–taker like Marge, who has Spina Bifida, that is a major achievement.

Marge was born in 1947 at the Cleveland Clinic in Ohio. The doctors told her parents, Mary Louise and Francis Hays, that their little daughter would be mentally retarded and would never walk– if she lived. After explaining her medical problems, the doctors recommended that the family leave the baby at the hospital to die.

"Fortunately," Marge says, "my mother saw things differently! She took me home and expected me to live. And I did, and I do– with enthusiasm."

Her diagnosis included conditions secondary to Spina Bifida: a series of spinal and hip malformations, little feeling in the bottom of her right foot, and no feeling in her toes. She can't always tell where her foot has landed. Because of that, three toes were amputated after being damaged. At birth, Marge's vertebrae were fused to each other in a strange pattern. A couple vertebrae were fused, then a normal one, then more fusing. Now, in her older years, they are almost all fused together. She has no tailbone and only a partial right hip bone.

Childhood was difficult, not only for Marge but also for her parents and her sister, Mary Frances. She struggled to walk, since her right foot had no feeling. The doctors told her family that she must be protected from falling, because she had no tailbone. They put her into several layers of diapers to give her more padding and spent a great deal of time holding her hands as she learned to balance. Eventually she could walk unaided, which led to more learning experiences.

"I was expected to perform all the things a non–disabled child could do," says Marge. "I learned to put my own toys away, feed myself, make my bed, set the table and do other chores. "Mary Frances helped me a lot when I was young. She played with me, babysat me, towed me around the neighborhood in a little red wagon and, one day when I was about 5, she knocked a boy off his bike after he pushed me to the ground. As my Big Sister (she is 9 years older than I), she always watched out for me.

"At the end of kindergarten, the school wanted to hold me back because I couldn't walk on tippy toes or backwards. My mom went to the school and had a 'talk' with them about my disability, explaining it was a miracle that I was alive." Marge was promoted to first grade after that conversation!

The relationship between the sisters was not always amicable. "When I was a teenager, we had to share a bedroom and our schedules were completely opposite of each other. We fought constantly–I had to get up early in the morning and get ready for school, while she had to sleep during the day to be ready to work her night shift as a Reservations agent for United Airlines. Mary Frances's benefits from working 30 years with United allowed me to travel extensively, for which I am very grateful!"

Marge had some reading issues during her school years, despite being an avid reader. After taking remedial reading classes in elementary school and high school, she completed a Bachelor's Degree in Teaching, with a second major in Spanish. She added a Master's Degree in Elementary Education and an Education Specialist's degree in School Facility Planning to her list of credentials. Marge taught for 25 years in the Denver, Colorado Public Schools, one year in Lansing, Michigan, and recently retired as a Home Hospital teacher for the Cherry Creek School District in Denver.

Her mother, Mary Louise, searched for new and creative ways her daughter could complete her daily tasks. Marge was horse crazy and demanded a chance to learn to ride. Her mother found a stable that would teach her everything about horses from the ground up, hoping that she would lose interest after mucking out stalls. That strategy didn't work. Mary Louise finally had to agree with her strong–willed child and let the owners of the stable teach her to ride. She continues to ride to this day, even after a painful fall at age 67. "I shattered my clavicle and needed surgery, a plate, and seven pins. When I fell, my horse stopped immediately. She looked down as if to ask, 'What are you doing down there?'"

Instead of complaining or giving up riding, Marge posted a gratitude note on Facebook, thanking family and friends who helped her through the trauma. "I'm just glad I didn't slip on ice in the driveway and do the same thing. At least I was having fun at the time." That's a typical Marge Hays scenario–doing what she enjoys, despite the potential pitfalls.

Marge has been physically active all her life. "When I accomplish a challenge–physical or otherwise–I feel successful and confident. Why do I take the risks I do? I believe it's because I want to prove that I can do what people say I can't do. I want to prove others, and myself, wrong.

"I dated regularly and was married twice. I never had a boyfriend who was put off by my physical problems. My husband, Doug, helps me hike and I help him swim. I cook and clean, and he goes down the ladder into our crawlspace to get things from storage, or up ladders to paint. He does all the vacuuming because it hurts my back. We each do the things we can do. Our life is give and take, not just *take* because 'poor me, I have Spina Bifida and can't do stuff.'

"People have no idea how hard I work to look this good," she says with a smile. "I work out in a gym, using t–rex straps, planks, weights, leg and pull–down machines, followed by shooting hoops. I have one rest/relax day, one stretch and mobility day for balance and core work, two swim days, and one day to take a walk outdoors. "All this for an aging person with Spina Bifida," says Marge. "I'm getting stronger every day."

Despite constant struggles with insurance companies, government agencies, and medical personnel to get the help and support she needs as a person with a major disability, Marge continues to advocate for herself. Her insurance company refused to pay for orthopedic shoes because she doesn't have diabetes, citing Medicare rules. After fighting with Medicare for more than a year, she decided to discontinue her efforts when she was informed that the next step was Federal Court. Marge hoped to convince Medicare that Spina Bifida is a cause of neuropathy but was unsuccessful.

Travel is her passion. She has visited 46 states in the USA, including Hawaii. She has been to Spain three times, London twice, Mexico twice, both Canada and Switzerland once. She believes young people should try to travel as much as possible, even if they must go alone and borrow the money to do so. That is what she did the first time she went to Spain while in her 20s. It is her belief that travel opens your eyes to how other people think and live. It broadens your horizons.

"As someone with Spina Bifida, I learned early on that if you fall, you must get back up. Sometimes you're lucky and there is someone to help but usually you must do it yourself! This philosophy has helped me throughout my life and not just with the actual physical falls–of which there were many. It gets 'old' sometimes, with all the surgeries and other problems, but I don't believe in being bitter or whiny. Everyone in the world has some issue that causes them grief–we just might not be able to see it. My disability is more obvious.

"When I was seven years old, I fell and skinned my knees. As I cried to my mother about life not being fair, she took my little face in her hands and said, 'Who the $%# told you life was fair?' It was the only time I ever heard her swear. I got the point at that young age. Life isn't fair. That's not the issue. Life just is what it is.

"Although Mary Frances and I were always friendly, after our mother died in 1975, we became much closer. She was in a terrible car accident in her 50s–rescuers had to cut her out of her completely demolished car. Multiple breaks to all four limbs left her in a coma for 10 days and in the hospital in traction for six months. I have no idea how she survived all this. Since the accident, I have had more and more responsibility for her, even though I am in my 70s and she is an octogenarian–both of us getting closer to old age.

"I have a lot of control over what happens to me. Sure, I didn't ask for Spina Bifida, but I have it and all the issues it includes. I take what I have and go for it, no holds barred. I take care of myself. I do the things daily that I need to do to keep healthy, and that means a lot more than swallowing a bunch of vitamins.

"I don't ask others to feel sorry for me and help me all the time. My parents expected me to be all that I could be. They helped me when the chips were down. It was a great start, and I will always be grateful."

CHAPTER FIVE

Enterprising and Creative
Diane Glass

When I was born in 1947, at a hospital in Waterloo, IA, I was taken home to die since the doctor did not know how to treat me. My parents were traumatized by my diagnosis and pessimistic since another baby with Spina Bifida had been born that same week in that same hospital and died within days. When I was 10 months old, they took me to the University of Iowa Hospital to seek further treatment. At that time my myelomeningocele was closed–that was the good news; however, I was born with only one functioning kidney, a tethered spinal cord and a neurogenic bladder, all of which had to be dealt with.

My parents had two other children–my sister Eileen, who is five years older than I and my sister, Susie, 10 months younger. Susie and I played board games, card games, badminton and created our own games of search and discovery. We would ride on our bicycles from one end of town to the other. We loved to tease Eileen, who mostly ignored it, except when her boyfriend came over and we tried to listen in on their conversations!

At Christmas, our entire family made the holiday special in our own unique way. My dad played Santa Claus, delivering presents to our side door since we didn't have a chimney. Mother baked angel food cakes and Susie and I made cookies. We all decorated the Christmas tree–a real one of course–and opened presents on Christmas Eve. After attending Midnight Mass, we slept in on Christmas morning and then spent the day playing the board games we had received as presents. So, you see, I did "normal" childhood things with my family.

I was a good student in school but, as I progressed through the grades, I had to deal with some emotional and psychological issues. I was continually anxious about my bladder leaking and having to wear diapers; this held me back from participating in typical activities like field trips, going to camp and slumber parties. My parents did not have the tools or knowledge to help me deal with my anxiety, but I know they did the best they could.

I didn't meet anyone with Spina Bifida until I was in my 30s, at which time I became more aware of how this birth defect creates disabling conditions. I never thought of myself as disabled, and still don't since I continue to find a way around the obstacles that could prevent me from doing what I want to do.

Today, my health issues include neuropathy, chronic back pain, and growing leg weakness. Doctors did not know about tethered cords or decided not to talk about this problem until I was in my 30s. At that point they felt the risks associated with surgery outweighed any possible benefits. The tethered cord contributes to both my leg weakness and nerve pain.

I have survived not only Spina Bifida but also breast cancer. Still I don't think of myself as a survivor. I experience life fully and find wisdom and energy in working through illness. The opportunity to build community gives me life. I find community through small group activities like writing, spiritual guidance, dinner clubs, and participation in arts and culture.

I value belonging to something bigger than myself, a caring cosmos, which some might call "God." That propels me to serve however I can: on the board of the Spina Bifida Association of Iowa, in my church as a healing minister, for the local homeless shelter in providing meals, and with my grandchildren. I also support friends through illness and loss by making and delivering soup.

My husband, Jeff, and I are both primarily retired. My stepson, Aaron, and his wife, Saraswati, have two adorable children, Soma, 8, and Raadhya, 5. They bring diversity to our family and joy to our lives. Saras is from India and we join them in celebrating Hindi rituals. My other stepson, Tim, is deceased.

If I could be granted three wishes right now, these are what they would be:

...that Jeff and I be able to see our grandchildren graduate from high school and continue their education;

...that I be able to complete a book of poetry for my family that provides a sense of my values and life experience;

...that people with disabilities be fully integrated into the community, valued for the contributions they make.

Facing life's challenge is like dancing. We move back, we move forward, we go around what is in our way. Sometimes we leave the dance floor altogether. I have developed a rhythm for working with illness that keeps me vibrant and engaged. I may not always choose the music, but I find a way to dance to it.[6]

---

[6] Diane's memoir, ***This Need to Dance: A Life of Rhythm and Resilience***, can be purchased at Amazon.com.

CHAPTER SIX

It's Not Normal to Be Perfect
Victoria Sandoval De Lara
In cooperation with Dorothy Hill Baroch

Born in 1975 with Spina Bifida, Victoria Sandoval De Lara, never thought of herself as a girl with a disability.

"I always knew that I have Spina Bifida, but never did I see it as something that can stop me from doing what I decide to do. In explaining my situation, my mother made things seem so simple. She told me that some people wear glasses, some use hearing aids, others use braces, like I do. She reminded me that everyone is unique.

"I attended an all–girls' school in Guatemala City where we had to wear a uniform. My mother didn't allow me to wear the skirt," said Vicky, "because I don't have any sensation from my knees to my toes. So, if I fell down (which happened often), I would hurt myself and not realize it until someone screamed that I was bleeding. Instead, my mother insisted that I wear pants of the same fabric as the skirt to protect me if I had a fall. The pants were not beautiful, and I did not like having to wear them, but her explanation helped me understand and made it easier for me to accept wearing something different than my friends.

"That simplicity allowed me to explain the situation to my peers, and they were satisfied with the explanation. Surprisingly, some of my friends from school now tell me that they were jealous that I could wear pants and they could not."

"Mother would not let my siblings and me say, 'I can't do that' so we always had to find a way to accomplish what sometimes was difficult for us."

Those are some of the factors that encouraged Vicky to be the person she is today. After finishing high school, the next step was going to University, with the goal of becoming an attorney. She accomplished that goal and now practices as a corporate attorney, also practicing criminal and labor law.

In 2007, Vicky and Jorge Lara were married. They have two children–Martin, born in 2009 and Agustina, born in 2011. Jorge is in engineering, works in telecommunication, and teaches at the University in Guatemala City.

In early 2000 Vicky became aware of a unique civil rights situation in her country and in 2018 she appeared before the Helsinki Commission at a United States Congressional hearing in Washington, D. C. She advocated for a Russian family, living in Guatemala City, who were victims of Russian political persecution because they would not accept the government's invitations to participate in corruption schemes.

Another aspect of Vicky's life has been her involvement in developing an organization in Guatemala that could address some of the needs of young people and children with Spina Bifida. Vicky and her mother were aware of other young people and children with the same disability, but most of them were not able to have access to good medical treatment. At that time, in the 1990s, many doctors in Guatemala thought it was better to let babies with Spina Bifida die. So, with other families impacted by the problem, they started AGEB, the Guatemalan Spina Bifida Association.

Trying to find the then newest information about Spina Bifida, looking for various treatments and hospitals and doctors willing to cooperate with their goals, the AGEB founders discovered more resources than they originally thought were available. People from the United States and Canada, Rotary Clubs in Guatemala and Washington state, doctors in Maryland and Guatemala, all helped the new organization to grow in many different areas.

"All together we were able to let people know that a person with Spina Bifida has the same abilities and opportunities that any other person has," said Vicky.

"I believe," said Vicky, *"that if you see yourself as a disabled person, people around you will have that perception about you. But if you know that you have some physical limitations as any other person does and accept that fact–being happy with who you are–that is how others will see you."*

"So, when I see adults with Spina Bifida who received help from AGEB as babies, achieving their goals in life, I know that all the people that have worked in AGEB, in one way or another have touched many lives–they have left a love mark in others' lives. And what is life about, if not about love?"

CHAPTER SEVEN

Helmuth Antonio Leal Espana, AGEB
Guatemalan Friend and Colleague

"I met Tom Baroch in Minneapolis, Minnesota in 2005 at an International Federation for Spina Bifida and Hydrocephalus and Spina Bifida Association of America Conference. Knowing Tom changed my life and I found not just another friend but a partner. Together, we tried to influence the lives of many in Guatemala. He helped the AGEB (Guatemalan Spina Bifida Association) organize the first International Conference in Latin America. He and his family were a key part in making it happen. For many years, he came to his second country, Guatemala, and in conjunction with Transitions Foundation of Guatemala, Rotary Clubs and AGEB, developed programs that had a big impact.

"Writing about Tom is talking about Making the Difference. Small, big, it doesn't matter. Making the Difference is action. It is example. Tom was action and Tom was an example of how you can advocate for change and impact peoples' lives. He traveled the world, and never said, "I can't." I am truly blessed to call him my brother. We share many stories related and unrelated to Spina Bifida. Even in his worst days, he had a smile. Always in the painful days he was helping others. His dream of coming back to Guatemala is gone but the spirit he left in the streets of La Antigua, Guatemala, where so many times he fell, got up and kept walking, will survive forever. The Spina Bifida community around the world lost a son, but a legend is born in his honor, and all of us should follow his example. God bless you brother."

CHAPTER EIGHT

A Father's Perspective
Edmund Baroch
As told to Dorothy Hill Baroch

It was early Saturday morning, December 12, 1959. Startled out of a deep sleep, I felt my wife, Dorothy, giving my shoulders a vigorous shake. "Ed, *please* wake up. I'm having labor pains."

"Are you sure," I asked, attempting to open my eyes. "Do you think they might be anticipation pains, Dorothy, since today *is* your due date? Would it help if you tried to go back to sleep?"

That proved to be impossible for both of us. The contractions continued in waves until sunup. Apparently, we were on the verge of an on–time delivery!

After a call to our doctor's emergency number, we left for Albany General Hospital. The contractions persisted throughout the day–close together, then farther apart. So, we waited. Talking, napping, visiting with the nurses. I stayed at her bedside, except for an occasional snack break.

That winter–shortened day passed, and it was dark outside again. We each dozed throughout the night, in between nurses' visits. Early the next morning things changed, and the nurses wheeled Dorothy to the delivery room. In those days, fathers were not permitted to watch the birth firsthand, so a nurse directed me to a spot in the hallway, in front of the delivery room doors, where I could peer–on tiptoes–through a small porthole.

The birth took longer than I expected, but since this was our first child, I didn't have a reference point. Then, a flurry of activity, and the doctor and nurses crowded around Dorothy. Instantly, things got even busier. More staff came into the room. One of the nurses came out to insist that I leave the area and go to the waiting room. I assumed that I would soon see the baby and Dorothy.

Time dragged. I read every magazine in sight, drank more coffee, waited, and watched for the delivery room doors to open.

Doctor O'Neill came into the waiting room, looking stunned. He told me there was a major problem and that the baby might not survive. In a fog, I tried to understand his explanation. All I recall is that the situation was desperate. The baby had a life–threatening malformation on the spine that could cause death or serious physical impairment. The condition was myelomeningocele, the most severe form of Spina Bifida. I also recall that Dr. O'Neill said–very emphatically–"don't let Dorothy see the baby, and for God's sake, don't let her hold him. Bonding can happen in seconds and it will increase her grieving when she has to leave the baby." He suggested that we place him in an institution and go about the business of raising the rest of our family.

"There's nothing more for you to do now, Ed. Go home and rest. You're going to need your strength."

"I'd like to see the baby," I said.

"OK, but only through the window. We don't want to move him any more than necessary."

I walked down the hall to the nursery, still rather bewildered. The nurse showed me what appeared to be a healthy baby, wrapped in a hospital blanket.

How could we consider abandoning this child? He looks perfectly normal.

I felt confused, devastated, and angry; yet the doctor told me there was nothing to be done–a difficult situation for an engineer used to solving problems.

Dorothy was still groggy from the anesthetic when I saw her briefly, gazing at her with all the tenderness and love that I felt for her. Then I left for home.

The doctor was right. The next day was a whirlwind of activity. I visited Dorothy again and our meeting was bittersweet. My first concern was for her and how she had responded to the news. Her tears told me some of the story but, as we talked, I saw her determination to fight it out.

"What shall we do, Dorothy?"

"I don't know the next step, Ed. I just know that I want to take our son home."

"I can't abandon him either. Let's talk to Dr. O'Neill to see what we can do to help our boy."

My mother–in–law, Grace Hill, was on her way from Baltimore to Albany, Oregon, where we lived, to see her first–born grandchild, and I planned to meet her at the Portland airport. We had friends who would offer to do that for us, if I were to ask, but since Grace was not aware of the baby's situation, I wanted to have some private time with her. At the airport, we met, and I explained what I knew. Our conversation during the eighty–mile drive home was limited; each of us lost in our own thoughts.

We went directly to Albany General, experiencing a tearful time, but one tinged with hope. Dr. O'Neill had visited Dorothy, giving her some options. A specialist from Salem offered a course of action that might be helpful, including taking Tom to Portland in an incubator for tests and possible surgery. It was a long–shot, but one we decided to take–anything to save our son.

It occurred to me that I had not yet called my parents. I told them of the problems and what we planned to do. They were concerned and sad, and my mother wanted to know more details than I had–what, how, why? When I mentioned to my father that we had named our son, Thomas, there was a long pause. When Dad talked again, he was hesitant, as if he were trying to contain his emotions. After we finished the call, I remembered that he had lost a brother named Tom, who died in early childhood–and for

Dad, fate seemed to be repeating itself. A wave of sadness erupted in me and I hoped with all my heart that our son would live.

The next morning, I went to the hospital, and after a careful briefing from the hospital staff, I fitted a small incubator into the back seat of my 1954 Ford two–door, making sure that it would not fall in case of a sudden stop. Theo Jones, the wife of my boss and a retired nurse, had offered to accompany me and the baby on the trip. When she arrived at the Albany hospital, we talked a bit, and then began the most harrowing ride of my life. Once at Samaritan Hospital in Portland, it took a few minutes to find out where to go. Theo and I had a short interview with an intern, who would be one of the medical team members working with Tom.

During all of this, I was numb. Some people thought I was a man of steel. I was NOT! My psyche protected me from falling into a million pieces. I did what was prescribed, not even thinking for myself as to what should happen–just robotically reacting. Many years later, well into my middle years, it occurred to me that my stoic behavior during that crisis period was expected– from others and from me. Hear the hard truth from the doctor, take care of calling and explaining, drive to Portland twice in two days, nervously protect my new son from any driving hazards, get a short explanation from the doctor in Portland, and so on. No thought that I was two seconds away from breaking down in sobs. Strangely enough, I was not even consciously aware of it. Once I understood this, I became angry. Why so little consideration of me? Just do it. Big boys don't cry. (We don't let them.)

Having survived the crises of those early years, I pondered my new awareness and concluded that, insofar as I could fathom, my anger had gradually disappeared. Now, my concern is for the fathers who deal with similar situations. No wonder so many of them cannot take it and end their marriages–leaving mothers to do it all. Support groups around the country, such as those developed by the Spina Bifida Association[7], were not available to me. Fortunately, parents of children born with Spina Bifida since 1973, when the Spina Bifida Association of America began, have had opportunities to learn more about the disability and its treatment, to share their thoughts and feelings, and to reach out to others in similar situations.

I feel grateful for my faith and for my belief in the family unit. That, and love for my wife and son, kept me from leaving when things over the years became more complicated. However, we faced each challenge as a family, researching doctors, surgeries, and actions that would allow Tom, and eventually his brother and sisters, to live rich, full, and productive lives.

Tom joined the Colorado Spina Bifida Association when he lived in Denver, served as its board president for three years, and became a member of the national SBA Board of Directors. Appointed by the national association as the United States liaison to the International Federation for Spina Bifida and Hydrocephalus, he traveled to many countries as SBAs representative.

Tom passed away unexpectedly November 4, 2018, one month short of his 59th birthday. The cause of his death was a pulmonary embolism and was unrelated to either Spina Bifida or hydrocephalus.

Instead of leaving him in an institution, as suggested by our doctor, we took Tom home, loved him and cared for him, allowing him the freedom to grow and live independently. The result–a life that was a positive influence on people with disabilities, and their families, on four continents!

---

[7] https://www.spinabifidaassociation.org

PART TWO

STRUGGLES AND TRIUMPHS

**The secret of change
is to focus
all of your energy
not on fighting the old,
but on building the new.**

Socrates

CHAPTER NINE

Sin Wages
As told to Dorothy Hill Baroch by Jackie

This is a cautionary, scary tale about my demon, Compulsive Tempter. So much of it has happened to many others just like me. Take heed.

One day, when my friend and I were on the way to play Roulette, we met Tempter. He was a friendly fellow and seemed genuinely happy to know us. I noticed he was carrying what looked like a big money bag. "Can I come along with you?"

My friend gave him a very worried look and said she'd just remembered someplace else she should be. I said, "Are you sure? We've planned this for a long time and Tempter is such a friendly fellow. It'll be FUN!!"

But Tempter said he certainly understood and never mind, he'd see her again soon. My friend said goodbye, and Tempter chuckled soft and low as he took my hand.

I told Tempter I'd better go with my friend. He said "Hey, no problem. I'd rather hang out with just you anyway. In fact, I have lots of lucky cash right here and it's all yours to spend in the casino AND you can keep what you win!" So, he gave me the bag of money and I started to play. Tempter just watched.

Well, sure enough, I won $666 on the first spin. In fact, I won on the same number six times in a row. I was hot!

And Tempter laughed soft and low.

I lost the seventh, eighth and ninth bets and kept losing. Soon the bag of money, as well as everything I'd won, was gone. I flirted with Tempter and asked if he had any luckier money that he could let me borrow until my fortunes turned around. Said I'd be glad to pay him back with interest. He chuckled soft and low but wasn't smiling when he told me that I'd have to use my own money now. "No, I should stop then," I said.

His smile came back. I believed him when he said, "I'm fine with that. But, you know, I like being with you SO much! Why not play just a little bit longer and I'm *certain* you'll win enough to enter the high roller tournament. Don't worry! I'll bring you luck." His laugh seemed to be growing harsher and lower.

The rest of the next eleven hours are a blur. At some point, Tempter left me and so did every dollar I'd brought with me. I even emptied my savings account to keep playing. I lost that money too.

The next day I got a title loan on my car and headed back to the casino. When I walked in the door, I saw Tempter talking to a young couple and handing them a big bag of money.

I was close enough to hear him chuckle soft and low.

ೞೞೞ

Hello. My name is Jackie. I'm a compulsive gambler.

Ten years. From 1988 through 1997, I tried to burn down my life. "Oh, not consciously," was the lie I told myself when the crisis came. That's only one of thousands of lies about gambling. Who knows how many over a lifetime about everything else?

My game was Keno, not Roulette as in the allegory above. I didn't meet the "Tempter" in person. Though, trust me, I can still feel him sitting there at the slot machines while I lost and "won" and lost, and lost, and lost everything.

My story of compulsive addiction is essentially the same as every other story told in Twelve Step Meetings the world over. It hasn't ended yet and never will in this life. That's why I'm "recovering" instead of cured. But there was, thank God, redemption. What would save me was Grace.

No sophisticate me, it all started with the California Lottery, scratch–offs and Bingo. Having an addictive personality, I couldn't/wouldn't stop playing until I was broke.

After moving to Las Vegas, the lure of casinos, especially the friendly neighborhood place around the corner, was irresistible. I never got a payday or title loan but time after time, I cashed my $824 paycheck at the promotion desk situated strategically dead center in the casino. With few exceptions, I'd walk out with maybe $20 to $40. I cleaned out my bank account and savings, borrowed thousands from relatives including my mom, uncle, and my not–yet husband. All on any pretext I could make sound plausible. Unfortunately, they always believed me. Until the world imploded.

Typical of addicts, I'd been a manipulative liar since childhood. I became one of the best liars as the gambling progressed. I managed to conceal everything from my partner until there were only two dimes left. Not enough for another bet.

18 August 1997

No more options. As President of my service club, I needed money to get to a conference in California. Ron got suspicious when I asked for another loan.

"Are you gambling?"

"No." The ten thousandth lie. Then it tumbled out. "Yes," and for the next three hours, I broke his heart with my confession. I said I wouldn't go on the trip.

"Yes, you will. You know how I HATE being lied to." He handed me $200. "Go."

The next three days were shattering. Would he be there when I returned? What would I do if he wasn't?

I came back to our home to find him sitting where I'd left him. It was August 18th.

"Well?" was all he said.

"Ron, I'm so sorry."

His blue eyes were storming. "Jackie, I don't get how someone as intelligent as you are could do something so damn stupid." He paused for a long, terrible moment. "At least I didn't until I went to a Gam–Anon meeting. I heard your story again and again. Sometimes, almost verbatim. I found out there are Twelve Step Meetings all around town."

"I want to go," I said immediately.

"Okay, there's one tonight at eight." And he came with me! Despite how badly he had been hurt by my lies, this man loved me enough to forgive me. Grace.

I attended meetings once, often twice, a day for two weeks.

Ron had been having trouble swallowing for a while and on September 1st, he was diagnosed with esophageal cancer. His surgery was on the 19th. He was given less than a five percent chance of recovery and maybe six months at most. We were married by a judge in our living room on October 15th. What a sad, sad holy day.

During those two weeks before his diagnosis, we pledged to stay together, put the pain and lies behind us and go on with our lives. Grace is unearned, undeserved, unconditional love.

I was saved by the Grace of those who loved and forgave me for the heartache I caused them.

My husband died on the second of December 1998.

I have never gambled again . . .

CHAPTER TEN

Searching for the Light:
An Encounter with Alzheimer's Disease
Nancy Nelson
In cooperation with Dorothy Hill Baroch

"You have early on-set Alzheimer's disease," says the stoic man in white as he attempts to give me a hand-written prescription slip for Aricept. Astonished and railing in my inability to think clearly, beside me a daughter in tears, I dismiss the doctor by bending forward with extended arm, and firm hand held up, emphatically putting a stop to the paper transfer for powerful drugs. There is no question about my response. Our eyes connect, and I shake my head from side-to-side. It's way too soon—no, I'm not ready.

"See you in three months for more testing," doctor throws across his shoulder as the door clicks quietly, and the man in white is gone. Jenn and I stare at each other in utter surprise and total disbelief. *Even though my Dad died from Alzheimer's in 2002, I never anticipated being diagnosed with it. Never.*

Alone, with no verbal explanation, no pamphlets, not even a sympathetic ear and kind voice, we are left by ourselves, feeling very much on our own. Jenn and I remain in our seats, neither of us ready to get up and walk out, carrying the weight of our news as though nothing had changed. *Everything* had changed!

Or had it?

In the hushed room, thoughts and reminders crowding in like scribbled, indecipherable notes. Memories...how is it I can get into the car knowing where I'm going, and wham! suddenly, I don't! I deliberately pull up to a curb close-by, giving myself time to recall the connecting streets to where I'm heading. Sometimes it takes only a minute, sometimes much longer. Memories...being on a bike ride with a close friend and couldn't find my own children's house on a familiar street in a familiar community. Memories...a Spanish class where I couldn't repeat words from my noggin' to just three inches down and out of my mouth. Memories...how I stood in front of a business networking group, ready to speak before a group of fifty, and I could not. Memories...how I meet you today and tomorrow will likely not know your name, recognize your face nor the content of our conversation. Remembering...how I forget business appointments or, one time specifically, a dinner date with dear friends. I leave them sitting in a fine dining restaurant—a no call, no show. When I realized, my stomach plummeted, and with a hung head and profuse apologies, I made an afternoon appointment and went to see her, for cancer was taking its toll and I was terribly disappointed in myself for missing our dinner date. She passed away the day after. I've never forgiven myself for time lost but honor her in a poem in my book. I live...with anxiety and frustration entering in and out of my daily life in tipsy, turvy sorta ways. It's been going on for a long time. Hard to fathom I didn't take real notice before!

Outside the doctor's office in the car, tears roll down my cheeks. Jenn and I cry, and we hug. Being very much her mother, I try to lighten our drive time home by saying, "What the heck!? It'll be okay." It didn't work. We squeeze hands, continuing down the hill toward the freeway, driving in near silence. In subsequent days and weeks, we were more reserved than usual.

Then time to sit down with my eldest daughter, Michelle, to explain what I really didn't know much about other than how I'd been feeling. My understanding of the three-pound brain, the 24/7 workhorse in my head, and the diagnosis of AD, was for sure very little, if anything. Alzheimer's disease, my Dad, and now me, and how it might affect my family—I was about to discover. Michelle and I sat close. I could feel her warmth. I wiped her tears. I wanted to take the burden from her, but how do I do that? My couple of weeks to adjust had given me some leverage and courage and, with profound mother/daughter-love, I weigh my words.

My journaling for answers came by way of poetry, early mornings, each day writing my heart-fears away. Sometimes when I read my poems, I wonder "who really wrote these words?"

Thoughts jumble, words disappear.
Times mix up, promises go astray.
When I hear, *"Where are you?" "Are you coming?"*
Eyes water, stomach churns, humbled in disbelief.
I know I have done it again!

Do I stay home, cancel, quit?
Or fight for rite of passage through the fog?
Silently, I say, I am not what I appear.
I am sorry for what you see.[8]

I ask questions of myself and of others. Answers are vague from both sides, and I walk in contemplation of *what now?* I feel diminished somehow. Quiet. Taking time to think, inquire more, listen more, read and investigate possibilities, all primary to finding peace. I need peace and answers and a plan so I can bring my family and myself through whatever is before us. Securing some medical and scientific insight on a misunderstood subject like Alzheimer's disease seems a monumental task. The internet is as close as my home office and computer, and I'm on it. I visit three different doctors and spend an inordinate amount of time dissecting what's being said, which means I should be figuring this disease out. Why is it then that I'm becoming more and more

---

[8] Excerpt from ***Blue.River.Apple.***

sketchy about how to deal positively with such a diagnosis or find the proper solutions to eradicate reasons causing brain cells to die and slough off. Can it be true that the medical profession really doesn't know? What I know is that it's tiring but I'm not giving up. I'm like a ravenous dog with a bone.

During this time, and still today, my eyes are wide awake most mornings before 5:00 a.m. Words and phrases showing up in my head and I still write them down on a yellow-lined pad. Those words and phrases certainly coming from an infinitely far greater source than myself. It is as though I am absolutely possessed. Words. Poetry. Blop! Here ya are!

Journaling helps me, and that's what my poetry is to me, journaling. Writing down what comes to mind as fast as I can, never letting the pen rise from the paper. I always wonder if it helps to be writing in a pretty book, or special bound journal? In my case, a yellow-lined tablet works perfectly. Name the topic and don't stop until two or three pages are completed. Guaranteed by the end of your writing, some solutions are settled in your mind or new options appear, and insights are clearer to you. If not, keep writing. It is how I work my way through diminishing memory, frustration, hesitation, and fear. Thoughts pour out to an eager hand which holds my favorite pen (do you have one?), and words flow fast and furious. A newfound understanding and feelings of wanting to be of service come forth. A mission of joy to spread courage throughout the Alzheimer's land, for not only the ones diagnosed, but their family and friends, in-family caregivers, and professional caregivers also. Giving back to a need greater than my own has been my salvation and, hopefully, could be yours if you'd like.

Perceived images and impressions about this dreadful disease seem to invade each person differently and leave them in a mere image of who they once were. It shows no favorites. As of today, this disease cannot yet be prevented, cured, or even slowed…and it's called a disease with a long good-bye. Even knowing that, we must remember there is hope and we must stand in faith.

Diagnosis. Cold hard facts set in.

{Shipwrecked.}
{Body strong.}
{Brain, hole-y, unhealthy.}

I glimpse ahead.
Summer's going,
Winter's approaching.

The undeniable truth feels like
Mind's fading. The slap stings my face.
As hesitation sets in
And confidence wanes,
My landscape now stark and wintery,

How to prepare?

Push back the curtain of fear.
Open the shutters.
Search for the light.

A spark—hope, fascination, heart.[9]

I attempt to eat better and forego sweets. However, it's a chore to keep myself in check. Exercise more, keep socially active, say "yes" to invites when I may not feel like saying "yes." Learning to become a better partner in my own health and realize, oh-so-well, communication is key. To listen more and exchange ideas

---

[9] Excerpt from "Thirty Days In," ***Blue.River.Apple.***

and opinions is a win-win. I volunteer. Helping others has been an energy booster in keeping my mind busy learning about "self-help and how-to" perhaps survive AD, or any diagnosis for that matter. We all have a challenge of some kind in our lives—to make the challenges lighter is to make lemonade out of a lemon-y illness, diagnosis, family matter, death, etc.

The Alzheimer's Association, Desert Southwest Chapter, came to my rescue and I hold them near and dear. I'm serving on the Leadership Committee still today and was fortunate enough in 2015 to work on the National Early Stage Alzheimer's Advisory Group (ESAG). Now, as an ESAG alumni, I am ready to give support when asked.

I speak up and out for Alzheimer's advocacy—building awareness, reducing stigma and promoting Alzheimer's programs wherever needed, I also volunteer for Alzheimer's Nevada and Cleveland Clinic Lou Ruvo Center for Brain Health. I've taken advantage of support programs, as well as facilitating some, and highly recommend the confidentiality and uplift it provides people looking for AD insights. Seek them out. It keeps me busy, and certainly by helping others, my Alzheimer's diagnosis is a sunnier weight to carry.

With new technology and medical testing, I recently received a revised diagnosis of MCI, Mild Cognitive Impairment. Is it correct? Never having attached myself to the first diagnosis, I think it not wise to attach myself to this latest one either. I'm reminded not to discount the positive outlook and ferocious regime that has gotten me to where I am today—fighting a good fight against an Alzheimer's diagnosis. And perhaps that my never-ending faith and hope have curtailed some of the AD advancement; just maybe keeping me disconnected from owning any part of all diseases listed under the dementia umbrella.

I give heartfelt credit to my family for their wonderful support. I recognize that a great deal of my optimistic attitude and beingness extends to those I call my bonus kids and families. They've shared familial connections having been in and out of my home for many years. Lucky me—and the list continues to special professional colleagues, long-time friends and new ones met within the Alzheimer's world. *What would I do without them?*

My drive and focus is to think
Better. Clearer. Longer.

Is to smile genuinely and grasp tightly
Onto the littlest of moments we share.
To retain pieces of air between us,
And the wisps of time around us.
Everything is important.

I don't want to go, **I say,** I think, I mean.
But when the time comes,
What my words and eyes
Can no longer communicate,
My heart knows forever.
Let me soak in your special essence
That you may radiate through my aura
and feel that *you are not alone.*[10],[11]

---

[10] Excerpt from "To My Family," ***Blue.River.Apple.***

[11] Dorothy Hill Baroch, author of ***Moments of Victory, Moments of Change,*** claims no copyright interest in the ***Blue.River.Apple.*** *series*, which contains poems cited in this chapter. All copyright interest in the poems is being reserved by Author Nancy Nelson.

CHAPTER ELEVEN

Stepping Stones To Success:
The Stories of Diana Mack Polanco and
Lourdes Mack Polanco
As told to Dorothy Hill Baroch by their mother,
Nicte Polanco Mack

INTRODUCTION

Following one's dreams or those of loved ones is not an easy task. Unexpected challenges, stumbling blocks, and ignorance are often obstacles–especially in the disability world. The parents of Diana and Lourdes, young women with major impairments, always seek the best options for their daughters–looking for opportunities that would help the girls accomplish their dreams. The following is the story of one family, but it represents the hard road that many families face as their children forge through life, sometimes leading the way for others as they make breakthroughs in a world that doesn't always understand their needs.

THE STORIES

Diana, a former resident of Guatemala, lives with a condition the doctors in her home country alleged had no cure and no name. During the early years of her life, her mother, Nicte, and the toddler, were involved in a new–to–them world of therapies, medical appointments–and more questions than answers.

Immediately after her birth in 1997, Diana began to have health issues but Nicte, as a first–time mom, wasn't aware of the extent of those problems. Baby Diana had cat–like cries and the lack of suction reflex. She was fed with a dropper and a spoon the first week of her life. Over the months, Nicte noticed the difference in development between Diana and her young nephew born two months before Diana. The family began to worry. At 18 months, Nicte's mother said, "I think Diana is not developing properly. She doesn't try to grab the toys in front of her; she is not following them with her eyes, either."

Nicte and her husband, Marcos, took Diana back to the pediatrician who, in the past, disregarded their concerns about the baby. This time, the doctor paid attention. Comparing head measurements, the doctor realized Diana's head had stopped growing and urged the family to seek help from specialists.

For the next year and a half, Diana was exposed to every possible therapy available to them in Guatemala. They tried swimming, equine therapy, neuronet, Glenn Doman method, physical therapy, occupational and speech therapy. Most of this was done with the help of volunteer neighbors. The budget and lack of financial assistance programs in Guatemala made the family pay everything out of pocket, so the key was to take Diana to therapy once a week or twice a month and repeat everything at home, every single day, from 8 a.m. to 8 p.m.

Nothing seemed to help. Progress was very slow, and the family had no idea what they were dealing with. They were confused, discouraged, and stymied until an aunt invited them to California for a visit. Their horizons began to open.

For six weeks, Nicte and Diana toured early intervention programs in Southern California's Shriner's Hospital, ophthalmologists, and pediatricians–anyone who could help them find an answer to Diana's mystery illness. They returned to Guatemala with pamphlets, books, and resources. For a year, Nicte tried to re–adapt to Guatemala's reality–no resources, no help, no school. Nicte toured numerous preschools, both local and far from their home, hoping to enroll her in school. The answers were heartbreaking: "We do not accept kids like her; other parents will complain." Finally, one school decided to enroll Diana for a year. Nicte secretly watched the children through a fence as they were in the playground. "My daughter was isolated; they were baby–sitting her, not teaching her. She was not getting any specialized help." And so, the at–home therapies continued.

In July 2001, Nicte learned that a second child was on the way. When she told her husband, he was concerned–worried about how they would care for two children, especially if the new baby were to have medical problems. Nicte followed the best prenatal care regimen she could access, hoping to prevent any problems with their second baby. They discussed whether to leave Guatemala in order to provide Diana with special education. They also hoped to find answers to their many questions about her condition.

Nicte wanted to have the baby in Guatemala and then move to the United States, but Marcos was fearful. What if the new baby needed medical care as well? They decided to come to the United States for ultrasound tests to determine if any problems existed. So, instead of waiting for the baby to be born, they left Guatemala on Christmas Day, 2001, and stayed with family members in California. The results of the ultrasound tests were surprising, and contradictory to the evaluation in Guatemala. The fetus had Spina Bifida. The possibility of returning to Guatemala disappeared with that news. The priority was to set a date for a C–section and do surgery on the newborn.

Lourdes was born on April 2, 2002. To remedy the problems associated with her diagnosis of Spina Bifida and hydrocephalus, she had fourteen surgeries from birth to age seventeen–four shunt revisions because of shunt failure; the rest of the surgeries were orthopedic, spinal, and urological.

From 18 months to three years old, Lourdes participated in an Early Intervention Program for children with developmental disabilities, held at UCLA and coordinated by the Regional Center, funded by the State of California. When she was two and a half years old, the teacher asked Nicte to be more consistent with Lourdes' attendance, saying that regular attendance would improve her speech. That surprised Nicte, since Lourdes' attendance was good. The problem–the child was not talking in school. That came as a shock to the family because she talked non–stop at home. Observation, however, indicated that she only talked to the immediate family; when guests, and even close relatives visited, she stopped talking. Since she was still a client of the Regional Center, the family requested a behavior evaluation. They determined that the condition was Selective Mutism. Some weeks later, a behaviorist came to the home; then two came simultaneously. Every week they exposed her slowly to new people, gradually taking her to playgrounds and other areas where there were new groups of people. They provided more and more opportunities

In California, Diana continued with various therapies and services, both at school and at home, including Occupational Therapy (OT), Physical Therapy (PT), speech and behavior services. Nicte had learned in Guatemala that repetition, intensity, and duration are key components for progress, so she worked with Diana at home.

At age six, she finally began to speak. Before that, the family used sign language and PECS (picture exchange system), which consists of creating a Pictionary with real pictures or visual icons.[12] Now they have apps for that but, at the time, Nicte drew, colored, cut and laminated each one by hand.

At age 12, Diana was clinically diagnosed with Cohen Syndrome, following a previous diagnosis of Autism–a very

---

[12] With the PECS system, the student points to the image to get what they want or need. It stimulates the language area of the brain, so eventually the person learns the word.

common characteristic and, a possible indicator, of Cohen Syndrome.[13]

Two years later, she was diagnosed with Retinitis Pigmentosa–a degenerative progressive problem with no cure–and another consequence of Cohen Syndrome. The disease left Diana legally blind and, with that diagnosis, the school funded services for the blind, such as teaching her how to use a cane for the blind plus orientation, mobility, and low vision services. At age 18, Dr. Barbara Crandall from the UCLA genetics department, did a genetic test via lab work and the Cohen Syndrome was confirmed. Attending Cohen Syndrome conferences and connecting online with families affected by the syndrome helped the family identify most of Diana's needs and health issues. Following their attendance at the 2016 conference, the family was able to convince UCLA to administer a life–saving medication that helped Diana's chronic upper respiratory and skin infections.[14]

Nicte and Marcos continue to augment the therapies provided by the professionals. They try to expose their daughter to as many opportunities available to her as possible–visits to museums, trips, and contact with animals. Diana enjoys having people read to her (because she can't). According to her mother, she is a living encyclopedia who memorizes everything she hears.

She receives speech therapy and has some speech challenges. Her volume, articulation, intelligibility, pronunciation, and lack of eye contact are poor, and, after a year of audiometry tests, it was confirmed that she has some mild hearing loss which impacts her speech. She can only hand–write her name. No assistive device

---

[13] A clinical diagnosis indicates one matches most of the characteristics of the condition, without having a genetic testing confirmation. The doctor suggests what the problem *could* be.
[14] Diana has a condition called Neutropenia–low levels of neutrophils, a type of white cell, which often accompanies Cohen Syndrome.

can help her, even though the family tried several methods, technologies, and devices over the years. She can't understand phonetics, word formation, or math, and doesn't comprehend time or the value of money.

With all her challenges, there is the occasional bright spot. Nicte recently received a wonderful e–mail from Diana's teacher. "Today Diana came up to me and told me she didn't want to go to the park. She told me it was too hot and crowded. I asked her where she would like to go, she told me TJ Maxx. So today we went to TJ Maxx! So proud of her, her communication and her self–advocating!!!"

This is the same girl who, doctor after doctor said, would most likely never be able to talk or walk. "Some people told me to send her to an institution," said Nicte. "Well, she is proving everyone wrong. She never stops learning and even if her progress is way behind others, she is doing it. I can celebrate with her every little achievement because for me they are not little, they are miracles!"

As Diana was growing and tackling her issues, so was her younger sister. When Lourdes transferred from the Early Intervention Program to public pre–school, the family encountered problems with the school system. The school provided a nurse for her catheterization, but the nurse was not trained in behavior intervention. Lourdes' anxiety surfaced again because of the new environment. The school system wanted the family to choose between her nurse and behavior management; they would not pay for both. Following discussions and failed mediation, the family took the school to court for due process. The judge ruled in their favor. They were allowed to continue behavior intervention at school and could keep the nurse for catheters and mobility. This approach continued until she moved to kindergarten. By then her progress was substantial, so the behavior services were discontinued.

Schools provide services and funds based on eligibilities but, without an eligibility diagnosis, many students grow up without intervention. Selective Mutism, which Lourdes had, was not an eligibility recognized by the school district. To have this problem as a teenager is a recipe for disaster; the levels of anxiety can be so high that it can be compared to being on stage all your life. Nicte attended support groups for this condition. Nicte remembers thinking, "I can't fix Lourdes' mobility problems, but I must fix the talking. She must talk or I will have a daughter who can't walk and can't communicate."

To help eliminate Lourdes' Selective Mutism, the behaviorist left homework every week, such as having Lourdes ask for her own food at the restaurant, celebrating and praising even just a word spoken or eye contact made. Exposing her to different environments was also important. Arranging weekly playdates outside of school with peers from school built her confidence once she saw that peer in the classroom. Nicte was advised to read different material to Lourdes–social stories appropriate for her age level–stories about anxiety, making friends, resolving conflicts. They read before going somewhere, reviewed what they had read as they traveled, reviewed once more before any activity was started. They asked Lourdes questions and acted out scenarios, then put what they had learned to test in the real world. Nicte and Lourdes went out for breakfast weekly, reading social stories while they waited for their food and practiced manners. The wait staff knew her, so they were patient with her. Little by little she started asking for her own food once the environment was familiar to her. That skill was slowly transferred to other restaurants and stores.

Many challenges of inclusion and accessibility were faced during elementary school: no stairs to the nearest restroom, non–accessible restrooms, lack of transportation for fieldtrips, and no nurse for Lourdes. Because of an administrative error, there was no school aide for either Diana or Lourdes for three months, so Nicte had to fill that role. Once again, they filed for due process, won their case and, within a matter of days, both girls had a school aide.

Constant non–compliance by the Los Angeles Unified School District to the Individual Education Plans (IEPs) for the girls, resulted in Nicte reaching a point of mental and emotional exhaustion. The family decided to relocate to Santa Monica because of the Santa Monica School District's reputation in Special Ed compliance, and because the family outgrew the small, non–accessible apartment in which they had lived for 10 years. They found an accessible apartment which allowed Lourdes to learn more life skills and to rely less on someone else's help.

There were some minor challenges with the Santa Monica School District, but nothing compared to the level of stress in Los Angeles. After a few years, the family requested an evaluation for their daughter. The conclusions allowed the IEP to be modified to implement techniques for her to cope with the issues that became evident during the evaluation process. Those issues included executive function disorder[15]–a common problem that affects people with Spina Bifida and which can be perceived as laziness or lack of interest. In the 7th grade, Lourdes felt she no longer needed an aide and that service was eliminated, allowing her more freedom of movement and more social interactions. Inclusion and creating friendships were on–going problems, but her love of theater was her salvation.

Lourdes was only four years old when she asked her mother to enroll her in theater. It was a challenge to locate an organization

---

[15]Executive functioning refers to the cognitive and mental abilities that help people engage in goal–directed action. They direct actions, control behavior, and motivate us to achieve our goals and prepare for future events. People with executive function disorder (EFD) struggle to organize and regulate their behavior in ways that will help them accomplish long–term goals.

that would accept her because, as some said, "we are not properly trained for her needs." Other companies did not offer to help with her accessibility needs. Eventually, Nicte found a theatrical company that was open to working with Lourdes. They provided a small ramp for her and if they encountered a problem, figured out what was needed. She worked with that company from ages six to twelve, when she could no longer navigate the stairs.

When she was seven years old, a non–profit organization made the family aware that The Joffrey Ballet was looking for a girl or boy in a wheelchair for the seasonal Nutcracker at the Dorothy Chandler Pavilion. Lourdes auditioned and got the role, working there for the season. At age ten, she auditioned for a role in the ABC drama series, Private Practice, landing a co–star role. She appeared in commercials and was a model for adaptive clothing. At age 12, she joined Infinite Flow, an Inclusive Dance Company, which she still attends. The company's mission: using dance as a catalyst to inspire inclusion and innovation, and to bring awareness to inclusion. She has been involved in multiple sports programs and was exposed to adaptive surfing, water skiing, tennis, rugby and wheelchair basketball. She was Little Miss Wheelchair California and appeared on the cover of Inclusive LA magazine.

In her first year of high school, Lourdes auditioned to be part of the annual musical and was accepted. This activity helped her make connections with other students and started to create a social circle. During the next two years, she became the first wheelchair user to become part of the dance class. This allowed her to complete her two years of physical education credits–doing something she enjoyed rather than being taken out of class for adaptive physical education. In her senior year, she continued with acting, studying Spanish, and is enrolled in college to study French.

Her involvement in those activities is a key component in her development as an independent person. Encountering challenges that often face a wheelchair user were not roadblocks to Lourdes following her dreams–they were stepping stones to success.

Nicte uses the same determination and loving care in helping her older daughter as she does with Lourdes. Diana earned her certificate of completion in high school and then entered an adult transition program, where she continues to learn life skills, the use of public transportation, money management, fitness, work skills and cooking. For the last three years, she has worked in a local store alongside an aide who trains her to complete tasks on the job. Through this program she continues to receive speech and occupational therapy and low vision services.

The steps to success are different for each of these young women, but they are moving forward on their own life journey– and accomplishing what others said was impossible.

CHAPTER TWELVE

Faith Reimagined
Molly Cowan

The story below demonstrates a moving example of a young woman re–discovering meaning in a faith she thought she had abandoned. Molly was raised in the Pacific Northwest for most of her life and currently resides in southern Florida. She is a recovering alcoholic with three years of sobriety and presently working toward pursuing her Master's degree in Clinical Social Work. She works as a client advocate and group therapist at a drug and alcohol treatment center for adults. Molly is passionate about helping others who are suffering and in the throes of addiction and mental illness, just as she was. She is especially interested in promoting social justice and advocacy for the underprivileged and underserved. She believes that those who have genuinely suffered can serve as a healing salve to others as no one else can.

"Being an alcoholic and suffering immense mental and emotional torture since I could remember, the crucifix had always represented pain. It represented a god that forgot about me. And honestly it seems that way for a lot of people like me, too. A god that didn't hear us. A god that let us and our families suffer, that "ruined" our lives. It was a god that wouldn't listen despite years of practicing militant–level devotion, prayer, and piety. I tried so hard to be good. I really did. But the pain continued and intensified. It didn't get better. It went on for years. And yet day after day I still went in front of God at mass, in confession, and in prayer, staring and begging at a god that, quite frankly, I grew to hate and despise. For years I looked at this symbol that represented that exact same emotional pain and alcoholic torture I endured and inflicted on everyone who ever loved me or tried to love me, especially my loving parents and younger sister.

Today, I realize that "god" was made up. That god wasn't GOD. That god was me. That god was a reflection of the things I had learned and grew to believe about myself and others. When I stepped back into the confessional through the Sacrament of Reconciliation after three years (one of the bravest things I have ever done besides getting sober), I told Him everything. I revealed the resentment, hatred, anger, seething guilt and shame, and horrible pain I had been carrying. I revealed my faults. All of them. Especially the ones I held onto. I left feeling empty. But it was then that I noticed slowly that the crucifix took on a new meaning. It now became a symbol and reality of mercy, grace, and incredible, literally undying love. I realized that God was with me, SUFFERING with me, the entire time. The E N T I R E time, even when I thought He wasn't. Even when I thought He left me to die. He heard everything. It was as if He had been whispering in my ear during those times, "Hold on, please hold on. I'm doing this with you. We're doing this together. I love you" and I was too blocked with self that I couldn't see or hear it then. And honestly, what is the point of a God who doesn't suffer WITH you? But I knew it was real. What the world offers as "love" is not the same. It's fleeting. It's superficial. It's unsatisfying. But the love of God fills my soul today. A REAL, living, and tangible God. Some of you will know what I'm talking about. And for that I am so so grateful."

APPENDIX

THOMAS EDMUND BAROCH
CAREER EXPERIENCE

Education

Certificate in Conventions and Meetings Management–Washington State University School of Business, Hotel and Restaurant Administration Program–**1993**

Associate of Applied Science Degree–Sous Chef–Portland Community College Portland, Oregon–**1989**

Professional Experience

- **Intern, Environment America, 5/2015–9/2015.**
Assisted the Clean Water Digital Campaign Coordinator on various projects.

- **Hospitality and Safety Ambassador Team Leader, Kiosk Hospitality Ambassador, Block by Block company, 9/2010–11/30/2014.**
Offered information and assisted people in the downtown Denver area who needed tourist information, business services, outreach, and other services.

- **Policy Intern, Colorado Nonprofit Association, 9/2011–8/2012.**
Assisted the Policy Director in monitoring and acting on local and national policies and bills that affect Colorado nonprofits.

Provided strong research skills on legislative and policy issues

Produced position papers, presentations, collateral material, and legislative action alerts in various media formats to provide information to CNA's members statewide

- **Events and Volunteer Manager, Autism of Colorado, 6/2008–8/2010.**
Led the agency in the planning of all fundraising, gala, medical conferences, family friendly events, and agency trainings and seminars

    Managed and worked with event and volunteer committees and third–party event organizers

- **Fundraising Account Sales Manager, Community Health Charities/Denver Employees Combined Campaign (DECC), 8/2007–2008. (Five–month contracted position)**
Assisted in the overall management of the 2007 DECC campaign, working with volunteers

    Arranged speakers and motivational events during the campaign for City of Denver department managers and employees

    Managed 33 City of Denver department accounts for the city's workplace giving program. Total raised: more than $564,000 in four months

- **Director of Development, Transitions Foundation of Guatemala/Asociacion Transiciones, Dual United States/Guatemalan NGO, 7/2005–12/2006. (Lived in Guatemala during that period).**

Managed the Development Department for the U.S. and Guatemalan disability rescue, independent living, job training, and education programs

Raised $700,000 internationally for Transitions through grant writing, corporate development, and individual giving

Supervised and made local arrangements for volunteers in the U.S.A. and those traveling to Guatemala to volunteer in–country. This included Rotary International clubs, church groups, and individual volunteers

- **National Catering Sales Representative, Boston Market Corporation, 4/2003–7/2005**

Sold catering packages and events to individuals and corporate clients for group meals, special events and corporate business meetings; increased product and services sales when possible to improve the bottom line of the event

Made daily cold and warm calls to develop more business for the company; contacted medical and corporate sales representatives as well as people who had called asking for information

Volunteer Affiliations

- Current Member: Steering Committee, National Council on Folic Acid (Since 2008)

- Current Member: Spina Bifida Association (SBA) (Since 2000)

- National SBA Board Member (2001–2004)

- Current Member: International Federation for Spina Bifida and Hydrocephalus (IFSBH) (Since 2002)

- Past International Liaison between SBA and IFSBH (2003–2007)

- Current member and past Board President: Single Volunteers of Greater Denver (2011–2013)

- Former volunteer: Metro Volunteers (2008–2012)

- Co–creator, developer, and occasional co–facilitator of the seminar <u>Engaging Volunteers with Disabilities</u>: Metro Volunteers (2008–2012)

- Member: Nevada State Assistive Technology Council (2018)

RESURRECTION

Diane Glass

Marble steps show shallow dips where footsteps tread down.
Dust motes float in filtered sun, descend on oak tables worn
smooth.
I pull heavy journals from library shelves, stiff board covers
nicked with age,
releasing dust, neglect, secrets, not opened for decades.

*The Journal for Developmental Medicine and Neurology
(1956–1962): one in 25 babies with severe Spina Bifida
not treated at birth survived after two years.*

In time, doctors drain fluid from babies' brains. But not 1947.
Take her home to die, doctors told my mother.
A ghostly glimmer of lost lives, dead for decades, chills the air.
The sun shifts, the room darkens. The clock nears five.

Something, someone saved me: luck, grace, love, God.
A restless mind searches for answers that soothe.
I pack up the past and ascend the time–worn stairs.
Sounds of students draw me to this summer day.

Dark and light intermingle on expanses of green.
Shadows of past and present come together.
Sadness companions joy, history yields insight, not answers.
Now the soul asks, free of certainty, wise to the heart,
not why are you alive, but how do you want to live?[16]

---

[16] Dorothy Hill Baroch, author of **Moments of Victory, Moments of Change**,
claims no copyright interest in the above poem. All interests in the poem are
being reserved by Poet Diane Glass.

CPSIA information can be obtained
at www.ICGtesting.com
Printed in the USA
BVHW050202100323
660169BV00011B/232